The Ultimate Weight Loss Hacks for Women of Any Age: Lose Weight, Feel Lighter, Energetic and Finally Take Control of Your Body and Physique

Debbie J. Wigington

Table of Contents

Chapter 1

Mindfulness Techniques to Foster a Loss-Oriented Mentality

It's difficult to lose weight. Snacking customs, unhealthy connections with food, and the ease of processed meals are all common obstacles to successful weight management. Though you may be surprised, the mind is more powerful than you may think. Eating well is more than simply making goals for the new year. It's good for your life, health, and overall quality of life all year long. Now let's look at some mental strategies to assist you develop a weight reduction mentality.

A Weight Loss Mindset: What Is It?

The capacity to think that you can and will reduce weight is the essence of a weight loss attitude. After the first burst of motivation fades off, our thinking sustains us. Weight reduction requires patience and time, as everyone who has successfully lost even a small amount of weight understands.

This implies that to sustain motivation over time, you will need to put in a lot of effort not just to lose weight but also to maintain the proper mental attitude.

1. Establish reasonable expectations and goals

Redefining your expectations in terms of what is attainable is the first step towards developing a weight reduction attitude. The environment in which we live has distorted our expectations due to quick satisfaction. It will be necessary for you to accept that true, long-term weight reduction is sluggish, uneven, and maybe even a bit of a chore.

Another thing to remember is that objectives must be specific in addition to being feasible. Trying to "lose 2 pounds per month over a year" will be much more effective than "losing some weight this year." You can create an action plan and see the end of the tunnel when you are concrete. On the flip side, not having a goal might just leave you feeling hopeless and overwhelmed.

2. Get Knowledge

Learning about the science behind diet and the newest exercise fads is another important step in changing your perspective on weight reduction. Believing you are eating healthily yet gaining a little weight may be quite discouraging. Thus, one of the most important steps in keeping the correct attitude is education. This isn't to give you a calorie obsession; rather, it's to give you the confidence that your hard work will be rewarded.

3. Let Go of the Scale Fixation

While it's important to track your progress and identify where you are beginning from, a common mistake made by many people is to weigh themselves once or more a day and bemoan the fact that they haven't made any progress. Weekly weigh-ins have shown to be quite helpful in weight reduction, according to Weight Watchers. However, weighing in more often than a few times each week may result in decreasing benefits.

4. Give up the idea that "foods are good or bad."

Speaking about unhealthful eating habits, the notion that you must abstain from certain meals may be too restricted for sustained success. Our triumph doesn't always end because we had a cookie. The reason for this is primarily because we consumed large amounts of "good foods" without knowing much more than what "good" and "bad" meant. For a diet that is nutritious over a day, week, or month, instead, strive to find a balance that you can keep to and that works for you.

5. Reevaluate Your Penalties and Awards

We all know, deep down, that motivation dwindles with age. Moreover, using a system of incentives and penalties is typical while attempting to maintain momentum. However, to what extent are the items we gravitate toward healthful? You're actively reversing your weight reduction progress if you celebrate your accomplishments with a slice of chocolate cake.

Furthermore, you will reinforce negative associations with food if you force yourself to work out for an additional hour after having too many drinks. This will prevent you from losing the weight you desire in the long run since diet and exercise will just seem like a never-ending punishment. This is not to say that you can't treat yourself to something special when you reach significant goals; rather, you should try to find incentives that have nothing to do with food or exercise.

6. Make thoughtful decisions

These days, mindfulness is all around us. It just means being in the now and paying closer attention to what you eat and how it makes you feel. This may be achieved via mindfulness meditations or even by just practicing being a bit more alert while making choices. Making mindful decisions may be a great way to change your eating habits, particularly if you're an emotional eater or a constant snacker.

7. Get Rid of the All-or-Nothing Mentality

Our tendency to think too black and white is another reason why we all give up on our weight reduction efforts a bit too soon. A healthy weight must be maintained throughout a lifetime; weight reduction is a gradual process. There will thus be ups and downs. You will sometimes get disoriented by your priorities. There will be instances in which you fail to act. Give yourself some grace rather than using such times as a justification to give up on the objective. Embrace the attitude that you will pick yourself back up the next day after every setback.

8. Take Your Time and Don't Rush Things

Research has repeatedly shown that sustained weight reduction requires a gradual approach. It may take months to drop the weight you need to reduce, even if you realize that losing 1-2 pounds per week is a healthy weight loss pace. Additionally, it will take longer if you weigh more. It's crucial to take your time making improvements. One area where slow and steady wins the race is weight reduction. Modify your perspective by emphasizing the adoption of healthful behaviors above achieving specific weight goals.

9. Remind yourself that you are in charge.

Recalling who is in charge is the key to developing an attitude that supports weight reduction. It's your life, and while it's simple to get comfortable and let the days pass by without doing anything, you are the only one who can lose weight. Take one action at a time to work on altering your thinking; you are in charge, so scale things up or down as necessary. Stressing yourself out is the last thing you should experience when trying to lose weight. When it comes to weight reduction, stress produces chemicals that may work against you, so take it easy when necessary.

10. Locate a Reliable Support Network

All humans are social beings. You may also maintain momentum by relying on a group of like-minded individuals to help you achieve your weight reduction objectives. Support for weight reduction is now widely available. Informally organized social media groups, commercial programs, online communities, and traditional gym companions are all available. Whichever strategy you choose, as long as you have support and someone to hold you responsible for achieving your objectives, it makes no difference.

The Verdict on Developing a Weight Loss Mentality

It requires more than just tracking calories and working up a sweat to lose weight. It takes a persistent mentality to maintain a healthy weight and lose weight successfully over the long run, even when your initial drive wanes. To make a significant difference, you must make several little adjustments, such as educating yourself and changing the way you see your weight reduction journey.

Chapter 2

Easy Dietary Tips for the morning

1. Get a big glass of lemon water to start the day

First things come first. Pour yourself a large glass of lemon water to start the day. Why? Your body goes into repair mode when you sleep, which involves a little detox. Moreover, you should drink some water since you went the whole night without drinking any. You may improve your "health" by including some lemon in the mixture.

Lemon water has many health advantages, including hydration, aiding in the liver's detoxification process, and maybe supporting normal bowel movements and digestion.

Extra benefit? Lemons are also a great source of important vitamins and minerals, including fiber, calcium, iron, magnesium, potassium, vitamin C, and B-complex vitamins. Vitamin C, on the other hand, is the one you should focus on since it is an antioxidant that aids in the body's defense against free radicals. That is to say, it strengthens your immune system and your skin.

2. Allot time for healthy breakfast

Your mother was correct! The most significant meal of the day is breakfast. mostly because being hungry makes it difficult to remain composed and in control of your situation. Additionally, having breakfast has a profound influence on the whole day, reducing your susceptibility to cravings and hunger later in the day. Breakfast provides your body with fuel and speeds up your metabolism.

Not enough time? If you have a busy morning schedule, you may prepare ahead of time by making something simple and fast, like overnight oats. Simply grip and move. But what happens if you have breakfast and your energy level drops in the middle of the morning? It might be the result of your choosing the incorrect proportion of protein and nutrient-rich foods. Your blood sugar is kept in check by protein, which maintains a steady level of energy. It also aids with fullness, which means you won't be grabbing for a sweet snack by ten in the morning (we all battle with that). Snacking on some nuts is a simple way to get some protein. Additionally, you may use collagen—a protein-rich morning supplement—in an omelet that fits the paleo diet or even a smoothie.

3. Commit to a five-minute prayer

Truth: You may feel a little... stressed in the mornings. However, did you know that even five minutes a day of meditation may help you stay healthy and focused? Entering meditation helps lower stress levels by promoting nervous system calmness. Additionally, when you start the day with a calm nervous system, your limited energy is directed toward other processes including digestion, mental health, and the brain (think concentration and attention).

4. Enhance your coffee experience

The most effective morning tip? Modify what you now do. similar to coffee. The collagen MCT coffee is the perfect pick-me-up that you can make by including some nutrients and healthy fats into the mixture. Your favorite coffee blend is combined with two additional ingredients, collagen peptides and MCT oil (also known as coconut oil). A supplement called MCT oil is promoted as the body's natural fuel.

Multi-chain triglycerides, or MCTs, are mostly made from coconut oil. Users vouch for the fact that it improves energy levels, mental clarity, and even heart and intestinal health. The flavorless Sproos Grass-Fed and Marine collagen mixes well with coffee, making it a simple method to get your recommended daily intake of collagen. Your skin, hair, joints, and stomach will all be grateful!

How to Prepare MCT Collagen Coffee

It's easy to make collagen MCT coffee. All you need is a blender, either a manual blender or an electric blender. To one cup of coffee, add one tablespoon of MCT oil and one scoop of your favorite collagen. Blend. You may add stevia or cinnamon if you'd like. You've been warned: MCT collagen coffee has a delightful, creamy flavor that may become quite addicting. It also helps to balance your energy levels and control blood sugar. Attention to detail, here you go.

5. Change your posture

Movement creates flow, and flow is always beneficial. Engaging in physical activity early in the morning helps to accelerate the body's metabolic functions, including digestion and metabolism. And these advantages continue long into the day. And don't worry about wearing yourself out afterward. The more energy you put into movement, the more energy you have. It's a "more is more" equation. It may increase your total energy levels, both physically and mentally, according to studies.

Which moving technique is the best? Your schedule may allow you to squeeze in a quick yoga session with your favorite YouTuber, or you may have time for a run or kettlebell class. Remember that every bit of movement matters, so whether you're riding your bike to work or doing a few stair sprints at home, movement is movement. And all of it contributes to getting your body ready for the day. Don't undervalue the importance of a healthy morning routine if you're planning to make improvements to yourself in the next year.

You may start the day as your best self by having a nutritious breakfast, drinking plenty of water with the additional advantages of lemon, exercising your body, scheduling time for morning meditation, and making a true health elixir out of your coffee.

Chapter 3

Easy dietary tips for the afternoon

Losing weight involves more than just nutrition and exercise. Making healthy lifestyle adjustments is only one of many sacrifices you must make to reach your weight reduction objectives. Many little things that we often ignore in our daily lives have an impact on how quickly we lose weight. You must thus be mindful of your everyday actions if you want to increase your metabolism and maintain your goals. Here is a list of the five-afternoon routines you should stick to remain on track and burn more calories.

Increase your water intake

It's common to mistake dehydration for hunger. Insufficient water consumption may cause feelings of hunger, irritability, laziness, and headaches. Therefore, have a long glass of water first to determine if you are really hungry or merely dehydrated before grabbing a package of wafers. You may also use infused water in place of your typical glass of water.

Enjoy your meal in silence

Your complete attention should be on your meal while you consume it. No monitoring of the Twitter feed, no answering to emails, and no browsing social media. You should not be distracted during the fifteen minutes you set aside for your afternoon meal. One of the greatest methods to avoid overeating and practice mindful eating two behaviors that are often linked to weight gain is to try this. For those who are attempting to lose weight, it is advisable to eat by yourself.

Observe your hunger

When you are overworked, it's normal to ignore your hunger pangs. Most individuals are unaware of the fact that this might eventually make you hungry, leading to overindulging at lunch. You must carefully prepare your food to avoid this. Eat little snacks to sustain oneself in between large meals.

Take caution while biting and licking

Again, watch out not to overindulge while you are eating snacks in between meals. Even if it may not seem like a huge deal to you, taking a bite off of your friend's sandwich or a handful of wafers will not help you with your weight reduction strategy. This will make you consume more calories during the day, which will undermine your attempt to lose weight.

Get going

After eating, consider going for a fifteen-minute stroll rather than just sitting down. Not only will walking after lunch help you lose weight, but it will also save you from crashing during the midday slump. Your mood will improve, your ability to concentrate will rise, and you will burn more calories as you walk more.

Chapter 4

Simple nutrition hacks in the night

1. Get enough sleep

The first step to optimizing your sleep for weight loss is to get enough of it. Sleep in and of itself can help aid in weight loss. "Sleep is necessary for normal body hormone and immune system function. A sleep-deprived or sleepy brain is a hungry brain," he said. "Poor sleep leads to weight gain."

2. Don't be a cardio junky

Cardio is great, and there are lots of good reasons it should be a part of an overall fitness plan. But strength training should be, too, especially for anyone who wants to take advantage of nocturnal weight loss. This is because strength training continues to burn calories after the session is over. A stop at the gym after work, or even a simple at-home strength workout can keep the body in calorie-burning mode all night long, even after bedtime.

Keeping a pair of dumbbells or a resistance band next to your bed is a good visual reminder to add in full-body strength training at least three times a week. Work the larger muscles, like the glutes and legs, as well as the arms, back, and core.

3. Do bodyweight exercises

Don't have access to a gym or dumbbells? Anyone can use their body weight to get in strength training. Do 10 squats before bed, followed by a holding plank for 30 seconds. Or try walking around the house one lunge at a time and then doing modified pushups on the knees for 5 minutes before hitting the hay.

4. Add hand or ankle weights to your walk

You don't have to give up your daily walk in favor of strength training workouts — simply pick up a pair of 1- to 3-pound dumbbells or strap on a pair of ankle weights to turn your walk into a strength training and cardio session in one. Since strength training is so important to building muscle and burning fat, squeezing a weight into your workouts when you can is a smart way to up your calorie-burning potential all day (yes, even when you sleep).

5. Forward fold for 5 minutes

Certain yoga poses help to calm and ease the mind of anxiety and tension. Try sitting upright in bed with the legs stretched out in front, then hinging forward at the hips. Feel a stretch in the backs of the legs (the hamstrings), and breathe in for five slow deep breaths and out for five. Feel a melting towards the legs and flex the feet. Perform this before bed to help calm down the nervous system and promote better quality sleep.

6. Sleep in a cooler and darker environment

According to a small study published in the journal Diabetes, people who keep their bedrooms at a steady temperature of 66 degrees for one month increased the amount of calorie-burning brown fat in their bodies by up to 42% and boosted their metabolism by 10%. A room that is too warm can also prevent you from falling or staying asleep. Bogan recommended setting your thermostat to 65 degrees.

To lose weight during sleep, try getting rid of that night light, too. Research suggests that light before bedtime can suppress melatonin and sleeping with a light on appears to affect the circadian regulation of metabolism, increasing the risk of weight gain, according to the Sleep Foundation. So, turn off your TV, phone and any bedside lights, and consider investing in blackout curtains to block light from outside.

7. Eat on a schedule

Charlotte Harrison, a London-based nutritionist at SpoonGuru, recommended keeping meal and sleep times fairly consistent. "Our body runs on a circadian rhythm, which is the 24-hour schedule our bodies use to help us to function. It's the body's internal clock," she explained. "Meal times have a lot of influence on our circadian rhythm, so scheduling our food is very important.

For example, if your body is used to eating between 6-8 p.m. then it knows when to prepare for incoming food by releasing the 'hunger hormones,' ghrelin and leptin, digest the meal, and then release the hormone melatonin to help us wind down for sleep. If we keep to the same rough schedule then our body can be prepared,

and we can get the most out of our meal and sleep times."
8. Eat a small dinner

There's an old saying: Eat breakfast like a king, lunch like a lord, and dinner like a pauper. There is some truth in it. Eating a big dinner too close to bedtime will take up your body's energy trying to digest instead of detoxing and recharging. So focus on a smaller dinner and a larger breakfast. And reserve your snacking for mornings and afternoons.

If you suffer from ailments like heartburn, eating a heavy meal before bed is likely to keep you up. "Even just the digestion process is enough to keep you awake at night," she explained. A recent study found that participants who ate a late-night snack broke down less fat than when they ate the same amount of calories earlier in the day. So, keep dinner light and small but don't go to bed starving either.

9. Don't drink before bed

Bogan suggested limiting your intake of alcohol and other substances as they can cause sleep disruption (not to mention easily adding a few hundred calories to your daily total). An evening cocktail may sound like it would be super relaxing, but even one alcoholic drink too close to bedtime can impede the body's ability to burn calories. This is because instead of focusing on burning fat as it should, the body is busy trying to metabolize the alcohol instead. So while a glass of wine with dinner is OK, leave it at that.

10. Eat protein all day long

Feeding the body protein every few hours helps stabilize blood sugar levels. And, this speeds up the metabolism all day (and night!) long. Protein is for building muscle, and it will fill you up, preventing overeating and the urge to graze on processed foods full of empty calories that can inhibit weight loss.

The body can only utilize around 30-35 grams of protein in one sitting. So if you're looking to build muscle, it's important to include it in every meal. Lean meats like chicken and turkey breast are always an easy go-to, and plant-based options like beans, quinoa, nuts, and edamame can help keep your meals interesting, while also adding a healthy dose of fiber (another important nutrient that fills you up and aids in weight loss).

11. Banish electronics from the bedroom

To lose weight overnight, all blue light devices, laptops, tablets, and/or smartphones need to go. Studies have shown that nighttime exposure to the blue light they all emit disrupts the production of the melatonin the body needs to promote sleep. In addition, a study conducted by researchers at Northwestern University reported that blue light exposure at night increases hunger and insulin resistance, which can, of course, lead to weight gain and not just the disruption of the body's fat-burning power.

12. Go to bed earlier

Aside from leaving you less time in the evenings to roam around the house and potentially snack, going to bed early can help ensure you get enough sleep. If you have a hard time falling or staying asleep, keep the room cool, dark, and free of electronics. As Bogan recommended, set your thermostat to 65 degrees and leave your phone out of your room.

Keep a book on your bedside table to help you unwind. By going to bed earlier, you'll ensure that your body has enough time to sleep and fall into your body's circadian rhythm, both things that contribute to weight loss, according to research.

Chapter 5

Simple workout tips to burn calories

1. Plank

- To begin, place your hands precisely under your shoulders and align your body so that your head and heels are in a straight line. This is the push-up posture.
- Keep your back flat and prevent it from drooping or arching by contracting your core muscles and maintaining this posture.
- Try to hold the plank for as long as you can; as your strength increases, progressively extend the duration.

An isometric exercise that works your core muscles and tones and strengthens your abs is the plank.

2. Mountain climbers

- Place your hands behind your shoulders and stand straight up to start the exercise.
- While in the push-up posture, alternate bringing your knees to your chest as if you were sprinting in place.
- When you keep your pace consistent, remember to keep your core tight.

A vigorous workout that increases heart rate, burns calories, and works your core muscles is the mountain climber.

3. Bicycle crunches

- With your elbows pointing out, place your hands behind your head while lying flat on your back.
- Elevate your head, shoulders, and feet off the ground.
- Stretch your right leg out while you bring your right elbow up to your left knee.

- Next, stretch your left leg straight and pull your left elbow near your right knee.
- Maintain this pedaling action while keeping your core active.

Exercises like bicycle crunches assist in toning your waist by working the rectus abdominis and obliques.

4. **Leg raises**

- Assume a prone position, keeping your arms at your sides and your legs extended.
- Lift your legs perpendicular to the floor while maintaining their straight posture.
- Lower your legs gradually back down so they don't contact the ground.
- To keep control of the movement throughout, engage your core.

Leg lifts strengthen the bottom portion of your core and train the muscles in your lower abdomen.

5. **Russian twists**

- Bend your knees and sit on the floor with your feet flat.
- Raise your feet off the ground and slant your back slightly while maintaining a straight back. While doing so, maintain your sit-bones balance.
- You may hold a medicine ball or weight in your hands, or you can clasp them together squarely in front of your chest.
- Rotate your body to the right and place your hands next to your hip.
- Take a step back to the middle and turn to the left.
- Keep switching sides.

Russian twists are an effective way to strengthen your core and develop your oblique muscles.

Maintaining a balanced diet and reducing abdominal fat are also important. To reach your objectives, you may combine these activities with a balanced diet and a comprehensive fitness regimen. For the greatest results, continue to remain consistent and progressively raise the intensity of your exercises.

Chapter 6

A simple method for burning calories

Cook at home.

Before your nutritious supper is delivered, spend forty minutes chopping, dicing, sautéing, and cleaning up your kitchen mess to burn off an additional 128 calories!

Dancing Party at Home

How can I burn more calories—roughly 107—without even realizing it? Play a dancing video game for twenty minutes, or simply dance to Lizzo in your room. Bonus: There's a strong possibility that you'll continue even longer.

At Home: Clean the Tub.

If you spend twenty-five minutes cleaning your home's restrooms, you can wave goodbye to soap residue and 107 calories.

Plant a Garden at Home

Plant a garden to improve your diet and burn an additional 105 calories per twenty-five minutes of digging in the ground. (Then use these clever storage tips to keep those fruits and vegetables fresher for longer.)

Express Your Creativity at Home

Wondering how to burn more calories when you're stuck at home? Shut off your computer or turn off the TV, then try painting. Try painting a fresh color in your bedroom or creating some art on a canvas. In any case, 35 minutes of brushwork will burn around 120 calories.

Get Dirty and Down at Home

Does the floor in your living room, kitchen, or bathroom need a thorough cleaning? You can brighten your house and burn 115 calories by cleaning them for only 15 minutes. (However, before you begin using this strategy to burn extra calories, have a look in your cabinets—some cleaning supplies may be harmful to your health.)

At Home: Peruse

Invest some time in a fantastic book, like these top sellers. Read for 65 minutes to maintain mental acuity and burn 100 calories.

At home, cut the grass.

Push the lawnmower across the yard to burn up to 119 calories in only twenty minutes when you step outdoors.

Hang pictures or paintings in your home.

Give yourself half an hour to hang the pictures or paintings you have lying about the home or in the back of your closet. In addition to saving money on a minor makeover, you'll also burn an additional 107 calories.

At Home: Give it your all

Take a 35-minute vacuum nap to eliminate an additional 100 calories.

For an added boost of functional fitness, try using your core muscles while pushing the vacuum as a way to burn more calories.

Stand Up at Work

To burn an additional 100 calories at work, stand at your desk for 40 minutes each day instead of sitting down. That's about as easy as it gets!

At Work: Take More Trips Across the Office

Go to your coworker's desk and ask a query rather than sending that SMS or email. Do you need copies made? Make them yourself by going to the copy machine. Going to the bathroom? Before entering, do one more circuit around the office.

All these extra steps add up. During your workday, an additional 40 minutes of walking corresponds to 119 more calories expended.

Workplace: Ascend the Corporate Ladder

You've probably heard this one before, but with good reason—one of the simplest, sweatiest ways to burn additional calories is to take the steps a few flights of stairs rather than the elevator. Stepping up for only 15 minutes throughout your workday will burn off 116 calories, or just three 5-minute walks. Not to mention, climbing stairs gives you more energy than coffee.

At Work: Arrange Your Workspace

Are you looking for ways to improve your emotional and physical well-being? Organize and tidy your desk for thirty minutes in the morning before you read your email. Simplifying your morning routine and getting rid of an additional 120 calories is a terrific idea.

Use the speakerphone at work.

To burn 100 calories before hanging up, put your morning conference call on the speaker (or use a headset) and walk about your desk or office throughout the 35-minute conversation. (Then step it up a notch with this best walking exercise for losing weight.)

Sneak in a little isometric at work.

To burn off around 100 calories before your lunch break, spend 5 minutes per hour before lunch doing some covert isometric exercises at your desk (e.g., squeeze your glutes and knees together and hold for 8 counts, then release). Replace your chair with a stability ball if your workplace is amenable to the idea. It won't give you toned abs, but it will increase your likelihood of sitting up straight and moving about more throughout the day.

Reinstate Recess at Work

To increase your energy and burn calories, grab some fresh air and engage in some interesting activities instead of having an afternoon coffee. In only ten minutes, jumping rope may increase heart rate, improve mental clarity, and burn around 107 calories. (Too much for your place of work? Get outdoors and remove at the very least. Just being in nature has many health advantages.)

Avoid the office candy bowl whilst at work.

Go ahead and relish those M&Ms if you are enjoying them. However, they're somewhat of a waste if you're simply mindlessly eating because you're tired or bored. Give up sweets (a big handful of M&Ms is approximately 100 calories) and you can easily cut down 100 calories or more throughout the workday.

At Work: Get More Angry

fiddling (tapping your foot, fiddling with your hair, etc.) may help you burn an additional 100 to 150 calories every hour, according to Mayo Clinic studies.

On the Run: Go Clothes Shopping

To burn off at least 100 calories, spend half an hour perusing the racks and trying on clothing at your favorite local shop or the mall (you don't even have to purchase anything!).

Always Have a Basket with You

How to burn extra calories when shopping for groceries: Take up a basket rather than a trolley and burn an additional 100 calories when shopping for 30 minutes. Because you'll be more likely to stay with the necessities rather than carrying about additional stuff you don't truly need, you could also spend less.

Stretch Away Calories While on the Go

Are you waiting for your food delivery or watching TV? To burn roughly 100 calories, do some simple yoga positions or stretches for 10 to 20 minutes. Besides, it feels nice.

Chapter 7

What is the ideal meal to eat to aid in weight reduction, and how can I lose weight safely and sustainably?

Severely calorie-restricting is not only not essential but also not recommended. Rather, eating full, unprocessed, high-quality meals is the healthiest and most lasting strategy to reduce weight. "These foods naturally raise your metabolism, reduce hunger, and encourage burning of fat," he explains.

Feit advises avoiding processed meals, fried foods, and refined sugars as much as possible. You should also be mindful of portion sizes. "The plate method is a great strategy; half of your plate should be fruits and vegetables, 25% should be lean protein, and 25% should be fiber-filled carbohydrates," she advises.

Eating a range of clear, unadulterated foods may also help your gut health. "Having a healthy gut can help reduce inflammation and boost immunity, which will improve your physical and mental well-being and help you stay on track to reach your weight loss goals. It also strengthens the insulin response, which reduces fat stored around the midsection," she continues.

Foods That Can Help You Lose Weight

The following foods have many health benefits that may help you lose weight and improve your general health.

1. Lean Protein

Lean protein sources like turkey, chicken, and grass-fed lean beef help control blood sugar, reduce cravings, and keep you satisfied. Legumes, beans, and lentils are examples of plant-based proteins that provide similar health advantages and increase satiety due to their high fiber content.

2. Eggs

Except for vitamin C, eggs are a good source of practically all the vital vitamins and minerals, including potassium, calcium, and phosphorus. According to Feit, eggs are not only a source of complete protein but can also be customized to suit a variety of palates.

3. Greens

Vegetables of all sorts may help with weight reduction. Broccoli, cauliflower, Brussels sprouts, and cabbage are examples of cruciferous vegetables that are strong in vitamins and fiber and may help ease digestive problems. On the other hand, dark green leafy vegetables are high in fiber, vitamins, and minerals as well as protein. Furthermore, low-calorie snack alternatives like celery and jicama are excellent choices for crunchy veggies.

4. Avocados

Feit claims that avocados are greatly underestimated. The fruit is an excellent meal for reducing hunger since it is strong in fiber and a good source of healthy fat. Avocados are high in calories due to their fat content, therefore it's crucial to watch portion sizes.

5. Fruits

Apples are rich in antioxidants and fiber. The fruit has vitamin C, polyphenols, and anti-inflammatory qualities.

6. Berries

Berries are rich in fiber, antioxidants, and vitamin C all of which your body needs to operate at its best.

7. Seeds and Nuts

Nuts and seeds provide distinct health advantages. All nuts reduce appetite and are a fantastic source of fiber, protein, and healthy fat. In the meanwhile, seeds are an excellent source of healthful fat and minerals. Here, too, watch your portion sizes. A quarter cup is the amount of nuts and seeds in one serving.

8. Salmon

Salmon is rich in protein and omega-3 fatty acids. According to research, omega-3 fatty acids may make overweight or obese persons feel fuller. Additionally, fish in general may make you feel fuller and more content for longer than other proteins like eggs and meat.

9. Crayfish

Shrimp increases sensations of fullness. By increasing the synthesis of cholecystokinin, or CCK, a hormone that tells your stomach when you're full, eating shrimp seems to reduce hunger. Moreover, zinc and selenium, two essential nutrients for a healthy immune system and more energy are found in shrimp and other shellfish.

10. Lupini Beans

Lupini beans are rich in prebiotic fiber, which nourishes the good bacteria in your stomach. The quantity and variety of bacteria in your stomach increase when it is well-fed. According to her, having a diversified and well-populated microbiome enhances gut health, which increases insulin sensitivity in your cells and helps burn fat that has been accumulated around the waist.

11. Raw Bananas

Unripe bananas are one of the world's greatest sources of prebiotic-resistant starch. Prebiotic-resistant starch increases insulin sensitivity in your cells, which helps to reduce the accumulation of fat around your waist. When paired with protein—for example, in a smoothie with nut butter and/or protein powder—it may satisfy your hunger for many hours.

12. Uncooked Oats

Resistant starch, or starch that resists digestion, is abundant in raw oats and is particularly beneficial for weight reduction. Resistant starch breaks down during digestion to generate byproducts that may increase insulin sensitivity in your cells and assist lose belly fat that won't go away.

13. Sauerkraut

Sauerkraut, or fermented cabbage, is a meal that is both probiotic and prebiotic, which means that it feeds the healthy bacteria currently present in your digestive system and introduces new beneficial bacteria. Additionally strong in fiber, sauerkraut helps manage blood sugar and hunger.

14. Vegetables

Legumes are good for intestinal health and satiety. Their high fiber content helps you avoid overeating by making you feel filled for longer. They also include nutrients that support the health of your gut flora.

15. Chia Seeds

Chia seeds may support weight management in two ways. To start, they contain a lot of fiber, which might make you feel full and stop overeating. Second, when you consume them unsoaked, they grow in your stomach, taking up more room and acting as a natural hunger suppressant since they expand in water.

16. Water

Even though water isn't a meal, it's nevertheless crucial for a good weight-reduction plan. Make careful to keep well-hydrated since all of our body processes metabolism is one of these processes that need water to function.

www.ingramcontent.com/pod-product-compliance
Lightning Source LLC
Chambersburg PA
CBHW071000250726
48663CB00002B/312